LIVING DAIRY-FREE

A Comprehensive Guide to
Managing Lactose Intolerance and
Thriving on a Lactose-Free Diet

Adams .U. Morris

TABLE OF CONTENTS

Chapter 1 5

Lactose Intolerance diet.............................5

Chapter 2 19

Lactose-Free Alternatives 19

Chapter 3 33

Building a Balanced Lactose-Free Diet........33

Chapter 4 49

Eating Out and Traveling with Lactose
Intolerance...49

Chapter 5 63

Coping with Social and Emotional Aspects ..63

Chapter 6 78

Long-Term Management and Future
Research 78

Conclusion...92

CHAPTER 1

Lactose Intolerance diet

Introduction: Lactose intolerance is a prevalent dietary issue that affects millions of people worldwide. It's crucial to understand the condition, its causes, symptoms, and how it impacts daily life. In this chapter, we will delve into the world of lactose intolerance, demystifying the science behind it and offering insights into its global prevalence.

What is Lactose Intolerance? At its core, lactose intolerance is a digestive disorder. It arises when the body has difficulty digesting lactose, a natural sugar found in milk and dairy products. Lactose, also known as milk sugar, requires an enzyme called lactase to be properly digested. Lactase is produced by the small intestine.

The Digestive Process: To grasp the essence of lactose intolerance, we must first understand the digestion of lactose. When a person without lactose intolerance consumes dairy, the body efficiently breaks down lactose into two simple sugars, glucose, and galactose, with the help of lactase. These sugars are then easily absorbed into the bloodstream, providing energy.

Lactose Intolerance Mechanism: In individuals with lactose intolerance, the production of lactase is reduced or absent. This means that when they consume dairy products, the undigested lactose reaches the colon, where it interacts with gut bacteria. This interaction causes a range of unpleasant digestive symptoms, such as gas, bloating, diarrhea, and stomach cramps.

Causes of Lactose Intolerance: Lactose intolerance can develop for several reasons, and it's essential to recognize its various causes:

1. Primary Lactose Intolerance:
   - This is the most common type and typically develops over time. As individuals age, their lactase production decreases. This explains why lactose intolerance often emerges in adulthood.

2. Secondary Lactose Intolerance:

    o Certain medical conditions, such as celiac disease, Crohn's disease, or infections of the digestive tract, can damage the small intestine's ability to produce lactase. This is known as secondary lactose intolerance.

3. Congenital Lactase Deficiency:

    o In rare cases, some individuals are born with a genetic mutation that impairs their ability to produce lactase. This is called congenital lactase deficiency, and it affects infants from birth.

Global Prevalence of Lactose Intolerance: Lactose intolerance isn't limited to a specific region or ethnicity; it's a global concern. Its prevalence varies significantly across different populations. Here's a brief overview:

- **Asian and African populations:** These groups tend to have higher rates of lactose intolerance, with some estimates suggesting that up to 90% of adults in these regions may be lactose intolerant.

- **Northern European populations:** In contrast, lactose intolerance is less common among individuals of Northern European descent, with prevalence rates as low as 5-15%.

- **Native American populations:** The prevalence of lactose intolerance varies among Native American groups, but it is generally higher than in

Northern European populations.

- **Mixed or diverse populations:** In countries with diverse populations, such as the United States, lactose intolerance can vary widely among different racial and ethnic groups.

This global diversity in lactose intolerance prevalence highlights the role of genetics and evolution in the development of lactase persistence (the ability to digest lactose in adulthood). In populations where dairy consumption historically played a significant dietary role, lactase persistence is more common.

Symptoms of Lactose Intolerance: Understanding the symptoms of lactose intolerance is crucial for early diagnosis and management. Common symptoms include:

1. **Bloating:** The accumulation of gas in the stomach and intestines, leading to a feeling of fullness and discomfort.

2. **Diarrhea:** Frequent, loose, and watery bowel movements.

3. **Gas:** Excessive gas production, often

accompanied by flatulence (passing gas).

4. **Abdominal Pain:** Cramping or discomfort in the lower abdomen.

5. **Nausea:** Feeling queasy or an urge to vomit after consuming dairy products.

It's important to note that the severity of symptoms can vary from person to person. Some individuals with lactose intolerance may experience only mild discomfort, while others may have more severe symptoms.

Diagnosing Lactose Intolerance: Diagnosing lactose intolerance typically involves a combination of medical history assessment, symptom evaluation, and diagnostic tests. Healthcare providers may:

1. **Review Symptoms:** Discuss your symptoms, their frequency, and their relationship to dairy consumption.

2. **Lactose Tolerance Test:** This test involves drinking a liquid containing lactose and then measuring your blood glucose levels to see how your body processes the lactose.

3. **Hydrogen Breath Test:** After consuming a lactose solution, your breath is tested for the presence of hydrogen gas, which is produced when undigested lactose interacts with gut bacteria.

4. **Stool Acidity Test:** This test measures the acidity of stool after consuming lactose. High acidity can indicate lactose malabsorption.

5. **Elimination Diet:** Some individuals may be advised to remove all sources of lactose from their diet to see

if their symptoms improve, and then gradually reintroduce lactose-containing foods to identify their tolerance level.

It's essential to consult a healthcare professional for proper diagnosis, as lactose intolerance shares symptoms with other digestive disorders, such as irritable bowel syndrome (IBS) or inflammatory bowel disease (IBD).

In conclusion, Chapter 1 serves as a foundational exploration of lactose intolerance. We've defined the condition, explained the digestive process involved, explored its various causes, and highlighted its global prevalence. Understanding these fundamental aspects is crucial for anyone dealing with lactose intolerance or seeking to support individuals with this condition. As we continue our journey through this book, we will delve deeper into strategies for managing lactose intolerance effectively, from dietary adjustments to emotional well-being.

CHAPTER 2

Lactose-Free Alternatives

Introduction: Now that we have a solid understanding of lactose intolerance from Chapter 1, the next logical step is to explore the world of lactose-free alternatives. This chapter delves into the options available for those who need to avoid lactose in their diet. We will explore lactose-free dairy products and various plant-based milk alternatives, as well as provide guidance on how to choose the right substitutes for your dietary needs.

Lactose-Free Dairy Products: Lactose-free dairy products are a lifeline for many individuals with lactose intolerance. These products undergo a process where the lactase enzyme is added, breaking down lactose into its simpler forms, glucose and galactose. This process effectively removes the lactose, making these products safe for consumption by those with lactose intolerance. Here are some common lactose-free dairy options:

1. **Lactose-Free Milk:** Lactose-free cow's milk is widely available in most grocery stores. It tastes nearly identical to regular milk and can be used in cooking, baking, and as a beverage.

2. **Lactose-Free Yogurt:** Lactose-free yogurt provides all the probiotic benefits of regular yogurt without the digestive discomfort. It's an excellent choice for breakfast or a healthy snack.

3. **Lactose-Free Cheese:** Lactose-free cheese varieties have become more

accessible in recent years. You can find lactose-free versions of many popular cheese types, from cheddar to mozzarella.

4. **Lactose-Free Ice Cream:** Enjoying a scoop of ice cream is possible with lactose-free options. They come in a range of flavors to satisfy your sweet tooth.

Plant-Based Milk Alternatives: For those who prefer to avoid dairy altogether or are looking for dairy-free options, plant-based milk alternatives are a fantastic choice. These alternatives are not only lactose-free but also suitable for vegans and individuals with dairy allergies. Let's explore some of the most popular plant-based milk options:

1. **Soy Milk:** Soy milk is one of the most nutritionally balanced plant-based milk options. It's a good source of protein and can be used in cooking, baking, and as a milk substitute in most recipes.

2. **Almond Milk:** Almond milk has a mild, nutty flavor and is low in calories. It's an excellent source of vitamin E

and is often used in cereals and smoothies.

3. **Oat Milk:** Oat milk has gained popularity for its creamy texture and naturally sweet flavor. It's versatile and can be used in coffee, cereal, and baking.

4. **Coconut Milk:** Coconut milk has a distinctive tropical flavor and is commonly used in curries, soups, and desserts. It's a good source of healthy fats.

5. **Rice Milk:** Rice milk is one of the most hypoallergenic milk alternatives, making it suitable for individuals with

nut allergies. It's a bit thinner in texture and has a mild taste.

6. **Cashew Milk:** Cashew milk is known for its creamy consistency and slightly sweet taste. It's great for making dairy-free cream sauces and desserts.

Choosing the Right Non-Dairy Substitutes: Selecting the right lactose-free or plant-based milk substitute can be a matter of personal preference and dietary requirements. Here are some factors to consider when making your choice:

1. **Nutritional Content:** Review the nutritional label to ensure the milk substitute matches your dietary needs. Some alternatives, like soy milk, provide more protein, while others may have added vitamins and minerals.

2. **Flavor and Texture:** Taste and consistency can vary significantly among milk substitutes. Experiment to find one that works well in your favorite recipes.

3. **Allergies and Sensitivities:** If you have nut or soy allergies, make sure to choose an option that

is safe for you. Rice or oat milk may be better choices in such cases.

4. **Cooking and Baking:** Consider how you plan to use the milk substitute. Some alternatives, like almond milk, work well in baking, while others may not thicken in sauces.

5. **Fortified Options:** Many plant-based milk alternatives are fortified with vitamins and minerals like calcium and vitamin D to mimic the nutritional profile of cow's milk. Check the label for fortification details.

6. **Sugar Content:** Be mindful of added sugars in flavored varieties of milk substitutes. Opt for unsweetened versions when possible.

7. **Environmental and Ethical Concerns:** Some individuals choose plant-based milk alternatives for ethical or environmental reasons. Research the production methods and sustainability practices of different brands.

Transitioning to Lactose-Free Alternatives: Switching from dairy to lactose-free or plant-based milk alternatives can be a smooth transition with a few practical steps:

1. **Gradual Introduction:** Start by substituting dairy with lactose-free options in one or two meals a day, allowing your taste buds to adjust gradually.

2. **Experiment:** Try different brands and types of milk alternatives to discover your favorites. Some may be better suited for specific purposes, like coffee or baking.

3. **Recipe Modification:** Modify your favorite recipes to accommodate the new milk substitute. With a bit of experimentation, you can often achieve similar results.

4. **Read Labels:** Always check product labels for lactose content and any potential allergens if you have food sensitivities.

5. **Seek Advice:** If you have specific dietary concerns or nutritional needs, consider consulting with a registered dietitian for guidance on making the transition.

In conclusion, Chapter 2 explores the world of lactose-free alternatives, providing a lifeline for individuals with lactose intolerance. We've covered lactose-free dairy products and a variety of plant-based milk alternatives, helping you make informed choices for your dietary needs. These alternatives not only offer relief from digestive discomfort but also open the door to a world of delicious, lactose-free culinary possibilities. As we continue our journey in this book, we will delve deeper into building a balanced lactose-free diet and navigating various aspects of daily life with lactose intolerance.

CHAPTER 3

Building a Balanced
Lactose-Free Diet

Introduction: With a solid understanding of lactose intolerance and a grasp of lactose-free and dairy-free alternatives from the previous chapters, it's time to explore how to build a balanced and nutritious lactose-free diet. This chapter is all about practical guidance, offering insights into essential nutrients, meal planning, and sample recipes to ensure individuals with lactose intolerance can enjoy flavorful and nourishing meals.

Nutritional Requirements for Lactose-Intolerant Individuals: One of the primary concerns for individuals with lactose intolerance is ensuring they receive adequate nutrition while avoiding lactose-containing foods. Here are some key nutrients to focus on:

1. **Calcium:** Dairy products are a primary source of calcium in many diets. To meet your calcium needs, turn to lactose-free or fortified plant-based milk,

calcium-fortified foods, and leafy greens like kale and collard greens.

2. **Vitamin D:** Vitamin D helps the body absorb calcium. While sunlight is a natural source of vitamin D, some people may need supplements. Fortified foods like cereals and certain plant-based milk alternatives can also provide this nutrient.

3. **Protein:** Lactose-free dairy products and many plant-based foods are excellent sources of protein. Incorporate legumes, nuts,

seeds, tofu, and lean meats or fish into your diet.

4. **Vitamin B12:** If you're following a vegan lactose-free diet, consider sources like fortified plant-based milk, fortified cereals, and nutritional yeast for vitamin B12.

5. **Fiber:** Ensure you're getting enough dietary fiber, which supports digestive health. Whole grains, fruits, vegetables, and legumes are rich in fiber.

6. **Iron:** Iron is essential for carrying oxygen in the blood. Pair iron-rich foods like

lentils and spinach with vitamin C-rich foods (e.g., citrus fruits) to enhance absorption.

7. **Potassium and Magnesium:** These minerals play vital roles in muscle and nerve function. Find them in bananas, potatoes, beans, and nuts.

Creating a Well-Rounded Lactose-Free Meal Plan: To build a balanced lactose-free diet, it's helpful to create a meal plan that includes a variety of foods from different food groups. Here's a simple guide to get you started:

1. **Breakfast:**

    - Option 1: Lactose-free yogurt with berries and granola.

    - Option 2: Oatmeal made with almond milk, topped with nuts and sliced banana.

    - Option 3: Scrambled tofu with spinach and tomatoes.

2. **Lunch:**

    - Option 1: Grilled chicken or tempeh sandwich with avocado and a side salad.

    - Option 2: Quinoa salad with chickpeas,

cucumbers, and a lemon-tahini dressing.

- o Option 3: Lentil soup with a mixed greens salad.

3. **Snacks:**

   - o Option 1: Sliced vegetables with hummus.
   - o Option 2: Trail mix with nuts and dried fruit.
   - o Option 3: Rice cakes with almond butter.

4. **Dinner:**

   - o Option 1: Baked salmon or a tofu stir-fry with broccoli, carrots, and brown rice.

- o Option 2: Spaghetti with a dairy-free pesto sauce and a side of steamed asparagus.
- o Option 3: Black bean and vegetable tacos with corn tortillas.

5. **Dessert:**

- o Option 1: Lactose-free chocolate mousse.
- o Option 2: Sliced mango with a sprinkle of chili powder and lime juice.

- Option 3: Rice pudding made with coconut milk.

Sample Meal Plans and Recipes: Let's explore a couple of sample meal plans and recipes to inspire your lactose-free journey:

Sample Meal Plan 1:

Breakfast:

- Lactose-free yogurt parfait with mixed berries and honey.
- Whole-grain toast with avocado.

Lunch:

- Quinoa and black bean salad with diced tomatoes, bell peppers, and a lime vinaigrette.
- A side of baby carrots with hummus.

Snack:

- Handful of almonds and a small apple.

Dinner:

- Grilled chicken breast (or tofu) with a side of roasted sweet potatoes and steamed broccoli.
- Mixed greens salad with balsamic vinaigrette.

Dessert:

- Dairy-free chocolate pudding with sliced strawberries.

Sample Meal Plan 2 (Vegan):

Breakfast:

- Smoothie with almond milk, spinach, banana, and a scoop of vegan protein powder.
- Whole-grain toast with almond butter.

Lunch:

- Vegan lentil and vegetable stew with a slice of crusty bread.
- A side of cucumber slices.

Snack:

- Rice cakes with cashew butter.

Dinner:

- Spaghetti with a dairy-free tomato and vegetable sauce.
- Steamed green beans with lemon zest.

Dessert:

- Sliced pineapple with a sprinkle of cinnamon.

These sample meal plans demonstrate the variety and deliciousness that can be achieved with a lactose-free diet. Experiment with different ingredients and flavors to discover your favorite lactose-free recipes.

Key Tips for a Balanced Lactose-Free Diet:

1. **Read Labels:** When shopping for packaged foods, carefully read labels to identify lactose or hidden dairy ingredients.

2. **Try New Foods:** Embrace the opportunity to explore a wider range of foods, including those from different cultures, to keep your meals exciting.

3. **Plan Ahead:** Meal planning and preparation can help you maintain a balanced diet and avoid last-minute temptations.

4. **Stay Hydrated:** Drink plenty of water and consider lactose-free or dairy-free beverages like herbal tea and coconut water.

5. **Consult a Dietitian:** For personalized guidance and

to ensure you're meeting your nutritional needs, consult a registered dietitian.

In conclusion, Chapter 3 provides a practical guide to building a balanced lactose-free diet. We've explored the key nutrients that individuals with lactose intolerance need to focus on and provided sample meal plans and recipes to help you get started on your journey to delicious and nourishing lactose-free eating. With the right knowledge and planning, it's entirely possible to enjoy a wide variety of satisfying and nutritionally sound meals while managing lactose intolerance effectively. As we move forward in this book, we'll delve into other aspects of living well with lactose intolerance, including dining out and traveling while avoiding lactose.

CHAPTER 4

Eating Out and Traveling with Lactose Intolerance

Introduction: Eating out at restaurants and traveling can present unique challenges for individuals with lactose intolerance. In Chapter 4, we will explore strategies and tips to help you enjoy dining out and traveling while managing your dietary restrictions effectively. Whether you're dining at a local restaurant or exploring far-off destinations, we'll provide guidance to ensure that your lactose intolerance doesn't hold you back from savoring delicious meals and memorable experiences.

Dining Out with Lactose Intolerance:

Dining out with lactose intolerance can be a delightful experience with some careful planning. Here's how you can navigate restaurant menus and enjoy your meal without the fear of digestive discomfort:

1. **Research the Menu in Advance:** Many restaurants now publish their menus

online. Take advantage of this by reviewing the menu before your visit. Look for lactose-free or dairy-free options, and note any dishes that can be easily modified to be lactose-free.

2. **Communicate with Your Server:** When you arrive at the restaurant, inform your server about your lactose intolerance. They can help guide you to suitable menu choices and convey your dietary requirements to the kitchen.

3. **Ask Questions:** Don't hesitate to ask questions

about ingredients and preparation methods. Inquire about any hidden sources of lactose in sauces, dressings, or garnishes.

4. **Customize Your Order:** Many dishes can be customized to be lactose-free. Ask for dairy-free alternatives like lactose-free cheese, almond milk, or coconut milk. Also, request that the chef omit any dairy-containing ingredients.

5. **Be Cautious with Cross-Contamination:** Cross-contamination can be a concern in restaurant

kitchens. Politely request that your dish be prepared separately from dairy-containing items to avoid accidental lactose exposure.

6. **Opt for Simple Preparations:** When in doubt, choose dishes with simple, recognizable ingredients. Grilled meats, steamed vegetables, and plain rice are often safe choices.

7. **Explore Ethnic Cuisines:** Ethnic cuisines like Thai, Japanese, and Indian often offer a variety of dairy-free options. Explore these

cuisines to discover new lactose-free favorites.

Dining Out Scenario:

Imagine you're dining at an Italian restaurant:

- **Appetizer:** Bruschetta with tomato and basil (ask for no Parmesan cheese).
- **Main Course:** Grilled chicken with pasta and a dairy-free pesto sauce.
- **Dessert:** Fresh fruit salad or sorbet.

Traveling with Lactose Intolerance:

Traveling with lactose intolerance requires a bit more preparation but is entirely manageable. Here are some travel tips to help you stay comfortable and well-fed on your journeys:

1. **Pack Lactose-Free Snacks:** Before you leave home, pack a variety of lactose-free snacks such as nuts, seeds, rice cakes, and lactose-free protein bars. Having these on hand can tide you over between meals.

2. **Research Dining Options:** If you're traveling to a specific destination,

research restaurants and grocery stores that offer lactose-free or dairy-free options. Apps and websites like Yelp, TripAdvisor, and HappyCow can be valuable resources.

3. **Learn Local Phrases:** If you're traveling to a foreign country, learn how to communicate your dietary needs in the local language. Knowing phrases like "no dairy" or "lactose-free" can be incredibly helpful.

4. **Carry Lactase Supplements:** Lactase enzyme supplements,

available over-the-counter, can help some individuals digest small amounts of lactose. Consult your healthcare provider before using them and consider carrying them as a precaution.

5. **Seek Accommodations with Kitchen Facilities:** If possible, choose accommodations with kitchen facilities. This allows you to prepare your meals using lactose-free ingredients from local grocery stores.

6. **Check Airport and In-Flight Options:** Many airports and airlines now offer lactose-free and dairy-free meal choices. Inquire about these options when booking your flight or while at the airport.

Travel Scenario:

Suppose you're traveling to Tokyo, Japan:

- **Breakfast:** Enjoy traditional Japanese breakfasts featuring grilled fish, rice, miso soup, and pickled vegetables, all dairy-free.

- **Lunch:** Savor sushi or sashimi without soy-based sauces containing dairy. Most Japanese restaurants offer dairy-free alternatives.
- **Dinner:** Explore ramen or udon noodle shops, requesting lactose-free broth and avoiding any dairy-based toppings.
- **Snacks:** Munch on rice crackers, fresh fruit, and edamame available at local convenience stores.

Portable Lactose-Free Snacks for Travel:

- Trail mix with nuts and dried fruit.
- Rice cakes with almond butter.
- Fresh fruit (e.g., apples, oranges, bananas).
- Lactose-free yogurt cups (if refrigeration is available).
- Nut or seed bars.
- Veggie sticks with hummus (if kept cool).

Remember, careful planning and communication are your allies when dining out and traveling with lactose intolerance. With these strategies in mind, you can embark on your adventures with confidence, knowing that you can enjoy a variety of culinary experiences while keeping digestive discomfort at bay.

Conclusion:

Chapter 4 has explored the art of dining out and traveling with lactose intolerance. It's a journey that involves research, communication, and thoughtful planning. By understanding your dietary needs, utilizing the tips provided, and embracing the culinary diversity of different cuisines, you can make dining out and traveling a pleasurable and worry-free experience. As we continue our exploration of living well with lactose intolerance in this book, we will delve into the social and emotional aspects of managing this condition and maintaining a positive outlook on dietary choices.

CHAPTER 5

Coping with Social and Emotional Aspects

Introduction: Living with lactose intolerance not only involves dietary adjustments but also emotional and social considerations. In this chapter, we will delve into the social and emotional aspects of managing lactose intolerance. We'll explore the emotional impact of dietary restrictions, strategies for handling social situations, and ways to build a support network that can help you navigate the challenges that may arise.

Understanding the Emotional Impact:

Dealing with dietary restrictions, especially those as pervasive as lactose intolerance, can have a significant emotional impact. It's essential to recognize and address these emotions constructively:

1. **Frustration:** Many individuals with lactose intolerance initially feel frustrated by the limitations it imposes on their diet. The inability to enjoy favorite

foods or dine freely at restaurants can be disheartening.

2. **Isolation:** There may be moments when you feel isolated, especially in social gatherings where food plays a central role. Feeling left out or different from others can be emotionally challenging.

3. **Anxiety:** Anxiety can arise from the fear of accidentally consuming lactose and experiencing digestive discomfort, particularly in new or unfamiliar situations.

4. **Guilt:** Some people experience guilt when they inconvenience others due to their dietary restrictions or when they have to ask for special accommodations.

5. **Acceptance:** With time, many individuals with lactose intolerance reach a stage of acceptance. They come to terms with their condition and develop strategies for managing it effectively.

Strategies for Coping:

Managing the emotional aspects of lactose intolerance is crucial for overall well-being. Here are some strategies to help you cope with these emotions:

1. **Education:** Learning more about lactose intolerance and understanding that it's a common condition can help alleviate feelings of isolation. Knowing that others face similar challenges can be comforting.

2. **Communication:** Open and honest communication with friends, family, and dining companions can make a significant difference. Explain your

dietary needs calmly and share your preferences and concerns.

3. **Preparation:** When dining out or attending social events, prepare in advance. Research menus, call restaurants to inquire about lactose-free options, or even bring your lactose-free dish to potlucks.

4. **Self-Compassion:** Be kind to yourself and acknowledge that it's okay to have moments of frustration or sadness. These emotions are natural, and they don't

define your overall experience.

5. **Support Network:** Build a support network of friends, family, or online communities who understand your condition. Sharing experiences and tips can be immensely helpful.

Social Situations and Peer Pressure:

Social situations often revolve around food, and dealing with peer pressure can be a challenge. Here are some strategies for navigating these scenarios:

1. **Be Proactive:** If you're invited to a gathering, let the host know about your dietary restrictions in advance. Offer to bring a dish that you can enjoy and share with others.

2. **Confidently Communicate:** When dining with friends or in a group, calmly and confidently communicate your dietary needs to the server. Most restaurants are accommodating and will do their best to meet your requirements.

3. **Dine Early or Late:** Consider dining at off-peak hours when restaurants are less crowded. This can make it easier to have a relaxed conversation with the server and reduce social pressure.

4. **Politely Decline:** If offered a dish that contains lactose, politely decline and explain your condition. You don't have to compromise your well-being to please others.

5. **Bring Snacks:** Keep portable lactose-free snacks on hand when attending events where suitable food options may be limited. This

ensures you won't go hungry.

Building a Support Network:

Having a support network can make a significant difference in managing lactose intolerance. Here's how to create one:

1. **Educate Loved Ones:** Help your friends and family understand your condition by sharing information about lactose intolerance and its dietary implications.

2. **Engage Online:** Join online communities or forums dedicated to lactose

intolerance. These platforms provide a space to share experiences, seek advice, and connect with others who face similar challenges.

3. **Supportive Friends:** Surround yourself with friends who are understanding and accommodating of your dietary needs. True friends will respect your choices and support your well-being.

4. **Support Groups:** Consider joining local support groups or organizations focused on digestive health. These groups often host events and

provide resources for managing lactose intolerance.

5. **Consult a Therapist:** If managing the emotional aspects becomes overwhelming, don't hesitate to seek support from a therapist or counselor who can help you develop coping strategies.

Success Stories and Testimonials:

Hearing success stories and testimonials from individuals who have effectively managed lactose intolerance can be inspiring and reassuring. These stories showcase that living well with lactose intolerance is entirely possible and can lead to a fulfilling life.

Here's an example of a success story:

"I was initially overwhelmed by my lactose intolerance diagnosis. It felt like I couldn't enjoy food anymore. But over time, I learned to adapt. I discovered delicious lactose-free recipes, found supportive friends, and even started a blog to share my lactose-free culinary adventures. Today, I'm not only healthier, but I've also found a new passion in

cooking and helping others with dietary restrictions."

Such stories highlight that with determination and a positive outlook, individuals with lactose intolerance can thrive and lead a fulfilling life.

Conclusion:

Chapter 5 explores the social and emotional aspects of living with lactose intolerance. While dietary restrictions can be challenging, they don't have to define your overall experience. By acknowledging your emotions, adopting coping strategies, and building a support network, you can navigate social situations and peer pressure with confidence. Remember, you're not alone on this journey, and there are resources and communities available to help you live well with lactose intolerance. As we continue our exploration in this book, we will delve into long-term management and future research on lactose intolerance, providing you with insights to support your ongoing journey.

CHAPTER 6

Long-Term Management and Future Research

Introduction: In the final chapter of our book on lactose intolerance, we turn our focus towards long-term management and the promising horizon of future research in this field. It's essential to equip individuals with lactose intolerance with the knowledge and strategies for sustained well-being, while also keeping an eye on potential advancements that may further enhance their quality of life.

Long-Term Management:

Living with lactose intolerance is not just about adapting to a lactose-free diet; it's about developing sustainable habits that support your health and comfort over the long term. Here are some key aspects of long-term management:

1. **Consistent Dietary Choices:** Continue to make lactose-free or dairy-free food choices that align with

your dietary preferences and nutritional needs.

2. **Monitor Symptoms:** Be attentive to your body's response to food. If you notice new or worsening symptoms, consider keeping a food diary to identify potential triggers.

3. **Regular Check-Ins:** Schedule regular check-ups with your healthcare provider to monitor your overall health and address any concerns related to lactose intolerance.

4. **Medications:** Some individuals may benefit from

lactase enzyme supplements, which can help digest lactose. Consult your healthcare provider to determine if these supplements are appropriate for you.

5. **Vitamin and Mineral Supplements:** If your diet is limited in certain nutrients, discuss the potential need for supplements, such as calcium or vitamin D, with your healthcare provider.

6. **Stay Informed:** Keep up-to-date with developments in lactose-free and dairy-free

products and recipes to maintain a varied and enjoyable diet.

The Promising Future of Lactose Intolerance Research:

Research in the field of lactose intolerance is ongoing, and future advancements hold the potential to improve the management and understanding of this condition. Here are some areas of research to watch for:

1. **Improved Diagnostic Tests:** Researchers are working on more efficient

and accurate diagnostic tests for lactose intolerance, which may simplify the process of identifying the condition.

2. **Tailored Dietary Approaches:** Future research may lead to personalized dietary recommendations based on an individual's specific lactose intolerance profile, considering factors like age and genetic predisposition.

3. **Treatment Options:** There's ongoing research into therapies that may help individuals with lactose

intolerance consume small amounts of lactose without experiencing symptoms. These treatments could provide more dietary flexibility.

4. **Lactose-Reducing Products:** Scientists are exploring the development of new lactose-reducing techniques for dairy products, potentially making them more tolerable for those with lactose intolerance.

5. **Probiotics:** The role of probiotics in managing lactose intolerance is an area

of active research. Probiotic supplements may help improve lactose digestion by promoting a healthy gut microbiome.

6. **Understanding Genetics:** Researchers are uncovering more about the genetic factors that contribute to lactose intolerance, which could lead to better-targeted treatments and prevention strategies.

Success Stories and Testimonials:

Success stories and testimonials from individuals who have

effectively managed lactose intolerance can serve as inspiring examples for others facing similar challenges. These stories highlight the importance of perseverance and adaptation. Here's another success story:

"Living with lactose intolerance pushed me to become more creative in the kitchen. I started experimenting with dairy-free recipes and discovered a whole new world of flavors. Not only did my digestive symptoms improve, but I also found a passion for cooking that I never knew I had. Today, I host dairy-free dinner

parties and share my recipes with others who face similar dietary restrictions. Lactose intolerance changed my life in unexpected and positive ways."

These stories emphasize that living well with lactose intolerance is not only about managing symptoms but also about embracing new culinary experiences and personal growth.

Staying Informed and Connected:

To stay informed about the latest developments in lactose intolerance research and connect with others facing similar challenges, consider the following:

1. **Online Resources:** Explore reputable websites, blogs, and forums dedicated to lactose intolerance. These platforms provide valuable information, recipes, and a sense of community.

2. **Medical Updates:** Regularly check for updates from medical and scientific sources to stay informed about the latest research findings and treatment options.

3. **Support Groups:** Consider joining local or online support groups focused on lactose intolerance. These groups provide a platform for sharing experiences and tips.

4. **Consult a Registered Dietitian:** If you have specific dietary concerns or nutritional needs, consult with a registered dietitian who specializes in digestive health. They can provide personalized guidance.

Conclusion:

Chapter 6 concludes our exploration of living well with lactose intolerance by focusing on long-term management and future research. By adopting consistent dietary choices, monitoring your symptoms, and staying informed about advancements in lactose intolerance research, you can lead a fulfilling and healthy life with this condition. The promising future of lactose intolerance research holds the potential for improved diagnostic tools, tailored dietary approaches, and new treatment options that may further enhance the quality of life for individuals with lactose intolerance.

Throughout this book, we've covered the fundamentals of lactose intolerance, dietary alternatives, meal planning, dining out, coping with social and emotional aspects, and long-term management. It's our hope that this comprehensive guide has provided you with valuable insights and practical strategies for effectively managing lactose intolerance and enjoying a satisfying and fulfilling life.

CONCLUSION

In conclusion, our journey through this book on lactose intolerance has been a comprehensive exploration of this common digestive condition. We've covered a wide range of topics, from understanding the fundamentals of lactose intolerance to practical strategies for managing it effectively in various aspects of life.

We began by delving into the basics of lactose intolerance, exploring the science behind it, its common symptoms, and the factors that contribute to its development. With this foundational knowledge, we moved on to discover lactose-free and dairy-free alternatives, both from the dairy aisle and the world of plant-based milk options. These alternatives open up a world of culinary possibilities for those with lactose intolerance.

In Chapter 3, we discussed the art of building a balanced lactose-free diet, emphasizing the importance of key nutrients, meal planning, and sample recipes to help individuals maintain a nutritious and delicious eating routine.

Chapter 4 ventured into the realm of dining out and traveling with lactose intolerance, offering practical tips for navigating restaurants and exploring global cuisines while keeping digestive comfort in mind.

Chapter 5 took a deeper dive into the social and emotional aspects of managing lactose intolerance. We explored the emotional impact of dietary restrictions, strategies for handling social situations, and ways to build a support network that can provide valuable guidance and understanding.

Finally, in Chapter 6, we looked towards the future of lactose intolerance management and research. We discussed long-term strategies for maintaining well-being and staying informed about the latest developments in the field. Promising areas of research, including improved diagnostic tests and potential treatments, were also highlighted.

Throughout this journey, we've shared success stories and testimonials from individuals who have effectively managed lactose intolerance, showcasing that it's possible not only to cope with this condition but also to thrive and find new passions along the way.

In closing, lactose intolerance is a manageable condition, and with the right knowledge, dietary choices, and support, individuals can lead fulfilling lives while keeping digestive discomfort at bay. We hope this book has provided valuable insights and practical guidance to help those with lactose intolerance live well and savor life's culinary delights to the fullest.

www.ingramcontent.com/pod-product-compliance
Lightning Source LLC
Chambersburg PA
CBHW060746260726
48660CB00002B/507